PROMOTE WELL-BEING NATURALLY

A natural neurotransmitter, serotonin is the secret behind such popular drugs as Prozac and "phen/fen." These drugs work by boosting serotonin's activity in the brain, thereby achieving their celebrated effects on depression and obesity. But serotonin does much more than modulate mood and control appetite. And there are safer, natural ways to restore internal peace, poise and self-control through diet, vitamin and mineral supplements and exercise. These approaches can be key to healing a remarkably wide range of neuropsychiatric conditions — from chronic pain and insomnia to Parkinson's disease and compulsive violence.

ABOUT THE AUTHOR

Syd Baumel is the author of the Keats book *Dealing with Depression Naturally* (1995). He has specialized in writing about natural approaches to healing and prevention since the early 1980s. His many articles have appeared in such publications as *Alive*, *The Aquarian*, *Bestways*, *Energy Times*, *Health*, *Natural Life* and *The New Age Connection*.

Serotonin

How to Naturally Harness the Power Behind Prozac and Phen/Fen

Syd Baumel

Keats Publishing, Inc. New Canaan, Connecticut

Serotonin is not intended as medical advice. Its intent is solely informational and educational. Please consult a health professional should the need for one be indicated.

SEROTONIN

ISBN: 0-87983-823-X

Printed in the United States of America

Good Health Guides are published by
Keats Publishing, Inc.
27 Pine Street (Box 876)
New Canaan, Connecticut 06840-0876

Keats Publishing website address: www.keats.com

Contents

INTRODUCTION

With quasi-religious devoutness, Jenny avoids every crack on the sidewalk, lest she "break her mother's back." Just six years old, she is already a captive to frightening obsessions, a slave to ritualistic compulsions.

Like his father before him, Jeff was a teenager when he took to drink and began his slide into mischief, violence and depression. Tonight—unemployed, desperate, drunk—he takes a rifle to his wife and children, then to himself.

Every day, Lydia has a new ache, a new pain. They keep her awake at night. They fuel her chronic fatigue and depression. Her doctors say it's all in her head—and it may be.

A massive body of research suggests these people have at least one thing in common: a deficiency or defect in the behavior of an important messenger molecule in their brains, a neurotransmitter called serotonin.

Of the dozens of neurochemicals that help mediate the complex comings and goings of our minds and behaviors, possibly none has come in for so much scrutiny as serotonin. It has a finger in almost every neurobehavioral pie: aggression, appetite, impulse control, mood, pain, sleep, sociability and more. Disturbances in the way brain cells called neurons use serotonin to signal other neurons—typically, deficiencies of "serotonergic" (serotonin mediated) activity—are proving to be a common denominator among a remarkably broad range of neuropsychiatric disorders. And drugs which boost serotonin—like the selective serotonin reuptake inhibitors (SSRIs) Paxil, Prozac and Zoloft—are proving to be the most versatile agents in the psychiatrist's little black bag.

Long before these medications became household words, a more direct means of boosting serotonin enjoyed widespread popularity: supplements of the nutrients from which serotonin is made. In hundreds of clinical trials, tryptophan and 5-hydroxytryptophan (5-HTP) showed that they often could equal or beat drugs at their own game. And while these supplements have druglike hazards of their own, it is becoming apparent that there are other, generally safer, natural ways of boosting serotonin: herbs, exercise, bright light and diet, among others. In this book we'll examine all these approaches, but first we'll see what the serotonin connection has to offer for so many of our aches and ills.

LISTENING TO SEROTONIN

As we are about to see, serotonin dysfunction appears to play an etiologic (causative) role in a very high percentage of diseases, disorders and minor upsets of the human nervous system. However, people vary tremendously: a generally serotonin-related condition can be highly serotonin-related for one person but entirely unrelated for another. Trial and error with at least one or two serotonergic approaches (one can work where others fail) is usually the only way to find out which of these groups a person belongs to. It's important to understand that most of these disorders can be related to other abnormalities (including other primary medical conditions) which respond to completely different therapeutic approaches. Depression, for example, often is a symptom of an undiagnosed illness, like hypothyroidism or diabetes (Baumel, 1995). While this book only focuses on the serotonergic approaches, you and your health care providers may need to cast a wider net.

MOOD DISORDERS

When it comes to the ups and downs of mood disorders, serotonin seems to play the role of mood regulator—a role which makes it a key player for some people, a bit player for others.

Depression

In the 1950s, the treatment of depression was revolutionized by two new classes of drugs: the tricyclic antidepressants (TCAs) and the monoamine oxidase inhibitors (MAOIs). Scientists soon conjectured that one of three powerful effects shared by these drugs could be the key to their success: boosting serotonin. A prominent British psychiatrist named Alec Coppen set out to see if serotonin's dietary precursor, tryptophan, could also work. It did, equaling drugs and electroconvulsive (shock) therapy in some trials. But it fell flat in other trials. Eventually, tryptophan gained a reputation as a weak or unreliable antidepressant, useful only as a booster of antidepressant drugs.

Nevertheless, Coppen's "serotonin deficiency hypothesis of depression" only grew stronger with time. Today, there is abundant evidence that deficiencies of tryptophan, serotonin and serotonergic brain activity are rife among depressives. With serotonin-boosting drugs like Prozac functioning like magic bullets for so many depressives, it is hard to understand how tryptophan could not be an antidepressant, too.

In the early 1980s, researchers came up with a credible answer. Tryptophan's poor showings, they noted, typically occurred when it was prescribed at a high dosage (van Praag, 1981). Perhaps tryptophan had a "therapeutic window," they reasoned, with too much being as ineffective as too little. Significantly, in most subsequent trials, tryptophan has continued to be at its antidepressant best at relatively low dosages of 2 to 6 grams (g) a day. Indeed, at much higher dosages, a contrasting property has emerged—tryptophan becomes a downer for people with mania. Tryptophan, it would seem, is fundamentally a mood regulator.

LISTENING TO 5-HTP

Years before Peter Kramer began "Listening to Prozac" (Kramer, 1993), a Dutch psychiatrist named L. J. van Hiele was paying rapt attention to 5-HTP, the intermediate compound between tryptophan and serotonin. "I have never in 20 years," van Hiele (1980) glowingly recounted, "used an agent which: (1) was effective so quickly; (2) restored the patients so completely to the persons they had been and their partners had known; (3) was so entirely without side effects; (4) failed so completely in about 50 percent of depressions. . ." (1980).

In roughly 15 clinical trials, 5-HTP has usually outperformed placebo (and tryptophan) or equalled antidepressant drugs (Poldinger et al., 1991). In the latest study involving 63 mostly severely depressed patients, it even outclassed the SSRI Luvox (fluvoxamine), one of Prozac's hottest rivals.

Bipolar Disorder

For depressed people with a personal or family history of extreme highs and lows—bipolar disorder, or manic-depression—antidepressants can be a blight, catapulting them into the minefields of mania or triggering a long, rocky course of rapid cycling from one extreme to another. For such people, mood regulators are the safest bet.

Lithium is psychiatry's preeminent mood regulator. But tryptophan is a mood regulator, too. Both these natural substances boost serotonin without boosting (like most antidepressants, including, to a slight extent, most SSRIs and 5-HTP) the brain's more stimulating neurotransmitters. In several studies, high doses of tryptophan (6-12 g/day), alone or in combination with lithium, have tended to rapidly bring manic patients down (Sachs, 1989). Indeed, some prominent psychiatrists have made tryptophan a staple of their mood-regulating arsenal (Chouinard et al., 1987).

ANXIETY DISORDERS

Research sends mixed signals about the relationship between anxiety and serotonin. While some studies suggest too little serotonin promotes anxiety, others suggest the opposite. As if to dramatize this ambiguity, serotonin-boosting drugs very often relieve anxiety disorders; yet they can initially exacerbate them, if not prescribed at a very low starting dose.

Serotonin boosters (SBs) appear useful for all anxiety disorders—from post-traumatic stress disorder to social phobia. Most clinical research has focused on the following major types.

Obsessive-Compulsive Disorder

People with obsessive-compulsive disorder (OCD) are plagued by disturbing thoughts they can't shake or by irrational compulsions they dare not resist—or by both. Until two decades ago, theirs was a notoriously hard-to-treat condition. Then along came Anafranil (clomipramine), a uniquely powerful SB. OCD and serotonin boosting have been synonymous ever since. Yet surprisingly little research has been done on serotonin precursors. In the 1970s, two of the original Anafranil pioneers gave seven OCD patients moderately large doses of tryptophan (3-9 g/day) with adjunctive niacin (vitamin B3) and B6. "The patients showed considerable improvement after one month of therapy, and after six months to one year. . .their conditions were stabilized," the doctors reported (Yaryura-Tobias and Bhagavan, 1977). But some of their colleagues later had no luck with tryptophan (Jenike, 1997). More reliable has been tryptophan's ability to markedly enhance the anti-OCD effect of serotonin-boosting drugs (Blier and Bergeron, 1996).

Panic Disorder

Serotonergic drugs are among the most effective treatments for recurrent panic attacks, or panic disorder (PD). So, perhaps, is 5-HTP. In one study, just 75-150 mg/day worked like a charm for 9 of 10 patients with PD and other anxiety disorders. Panic attacks as frequent as 45 a month all but vanished. In a larger follow-up trial, 5-HTP again demonstrated an antianxiety effect, albeit weaker than that of Anafranil (Kahn et al., 1987).

DISORDERS OF IMPULSE CONTROL

If there is a common factor in serotonin's varied roles, self-control may be it. People who are deficient in this virtue are apt to be deficient in serotonin (Linnoila and Virkkunen, 1992). And for them, a serotonin booster may be just what the doctor (or the parole officer) ordered.

Impulsive Aggression and Violence

One of the most consistent findings in all of psychobiology is the link between low serotonin in the brain and impulsive, explosive acts of violence (Linnoila and Virkkunen, 1992). It occurs uniformly in mice and men, in feisty chickens and scrappy alcoholics, in children who torture their pets and parents who massacre their children (Lion, 1995). In telling contrast, controlled aggression and assertiveness are associated with high serotonergic activity.

These findings are of more than academic interest. Serotonergic agents such as the SSRIs, lithium, progesterone, tryptophan, and 5-HTP have mellowed or pacified many a beast and many a beastly human (Lion, 1995). In

the lab, acute tryptophan depletion—and therefore serotonin depletion—tends to ruffle people's feathers, especially if they have a short fuse to begin with (Cleare and Bond,
1995). And in clinical trials, both tryptophan (alone or combined with the serotonergic drug Desyrel [trazadone]) and
5-HTP have helped juvenile delinquents, homicidal schizophrenics (Morand et al.,1983) and explosive, run-amok in-
patients (Watson and Philips, 1986) learn the meaning of
the word "chill."

Suicide
People commit suicide for all kinds of personal reasons.
But many studies suggest that, at least in the case of violent
suicide, there is usually a chemical reason, too: a nearly
empty tank of serotonin (Linnoila and Virkkunen, 1992).

Among people at grossly elevated risk of suicide—people with bipolar disorder or recurrent severe depressions—
long-term therapy with serotonergic lithium causes their
suicide rate to plummet (Müller-Oerlinghausen et al., 1992).
Even the lithium in some water supplies has had a statisti-
cal impact on suicide (Papaioannou and Pfeiffer, 1986).
And while SSRIs like Prozac may, paradoxically, have a sui-
cidal effect on some users, overall they markedly prevent
suicide, too.

Substance Abuse
One of the easiest ways to help strung-out laboratory ani-
mals just say no to drugs is to boost their serotonin levels.
In humans, too, there are signs that this strategy can work,
whether by boosting self-control, soothing withdrawal
pangs or simply scratching the itch that leads people to
drugs in the first place. Research has focused on only a few
major dependencies, but any could be fair game for the
serotonin solution.

Smoking
Boosting serotonin is one of many neurochemical effects
that likely account for nicotine's (killer) charms.

Acupuncture, which can also boost serotonin, quells the agony of tobacco withdrawal and rivals nicotine gum (Clavel et al., 1985). In a small pilot study, tryptophan (50 mg/kg) also curbed would-be quitters' withdrawal symptoms or cut their cigarette use significantly more than placebo (Bowen et al., 1991).

Alcoholism

Alcohol appears to satisfy a deep serotonin hunger in many alcoholics, only to mockingly exaggerate it should they try to quit (Buydens-Branchey et al., 1989). Yet clinical trials of alternative serotonin boosters—SSRIs, lithium, Buspar, 5-HTP—have usually yielded only modest and transient benefits for the average alcoholic seeking sobriety. Some researchers advocate targeting a not-so-average subgroup of alcoholics who show pronounced biochemical signs of serotonin deficiency. In true serotonin-shy fashion, these individuals typically are men with a history (like their fathers before them) of depression and attempted suicide, impulsive violence or other antisocial behavior and early-onset alcoholism. "Theoretically [these people] should respond to tryptophan supplementation or to treatment with other agents modifying serotonin functional levels," researchers speculate (Buydens-Branchey et al., 1989). Or to diet. As we'll see, they also are prone to reactive hypoglycemia.

OVERWEIGHT AND EATING DISORDERS

One of serotonin's functions in the brain is to put the brakes on eating, in particular of carbohydrates. In recent years, serotonin boosting has become the premier pharmacological aid in the perennial war on fat and compulsive overeating.

Overweight

As this book goes to press, the reputation of the weight-loss wonder drug popularly called "phen/fen" is being dragged through the mud yet again. First it was a rare, but deadly, complication called primary pulmonary hypertension. Then it was the little-publicized spectre of subtle damage to serotonergic neurons. Now, it seems, this combination of speed-like phentermine with the potent serotonin releaser fenfluramine may also cause heart valve damage in many users.

Too bad. Phen/fen and Redux (fenfluramine's stronger and similarly tainted sister, dexfenfluramine) have been magic weight-loss pills for many. Fortunately, research suggests natural SBs may work, too (although, as we'll see, their brand of serotonin boosting is also haunted by rare hazards similar to those of phen/fen).

In one brief trial, tryptophan performed about as well as phen/fen and Redux usually do, though the small number of participants made it fall short statistically of beating the placebo (Strain and Zumoff, 1985). The modest 3 g/day dosage probably had something to do with it, for strong serotonergic medicine is needed to curb appetite. Truly hefty doses of 5-HTP did outdo placebo in two studies by doctors from the University of Rome. In one, ten obese women lost 1.7 kg after six weeks on 300 mg 5-HTP, taken 30 minutes before each meal. When a low-cal diet was thrown in for the final six weeks, they lost another 3.3 kg, trouncing the placebo plus diet control group (Cangiano et al., 1992).

As we'll see, serotonin can also be boosted by dietary modification. MIT nutritionist Judith Wurtman finds this to be a potent weight-loss alternative to drugs (Wurtman and Suffes, 1996).

Bulimia Nervosa and Binge-Eating Disorder

Because high carbohydrate foods tend to increase brain serotonin, experts suspect that carbohydrate craving often represents an instinctive attempt to self-medicate their serotonin-related aches and ills. Certainly, people with the binge/purge disorder of bulimia nervosa often fit this bill. Likewise, their moods tend to deteriorate and their cravings flare, when they are acutely deprived of dietary tryptophan (Weltzin et al., 1995). At the Royal Ottawa Hospital, psychiatrists repeatedly turned one bulimic's symptoms off and on by prescribing and withdrawing a small nighttime dose (1 g) of tryptophan (Cole and LaPierre, 1986). In another trial, tryptophan was not significantly superior to placebo, but the placebo response was high, as often is the case with bulimia (Krahn and Mitchell, 1985). In further support of the serotonin solution, SSRIs are shaping up to be a treatment of choice both for bulimia and for its sister "bingeing-without-purging" disorder: binge-eating disorder.

PAIN AND INSOMNIA

One of the functions of serotonergic neurons is to muffle the din of incoming pain signals. Another, it would seem, is to dull our sensitivity to the stimuli that would otherwise keep us awake at night.

Pain

Since the 1980s, researchers have demonstrated the value of tryptophan for chronic pain in several placebo-controlled trials (Pollack,1986). 5-HTP has also shown considerable promise as a treatment for migraine headaches and fibromyalgia, a syndrome of chronic muscle pain and tenderness, fatigue and depression. In one trial 5-HTP beat placebo; in another it brought mild to marked improvements within two weeks to half of 50 fibromyalgia patients (Puttini and Caruso, 1992).

Insomnia

In the 1990s, melatonin inherited the "most-favored natural sleeping pill" crown once worn so proudly by tryptophan in the 1980s. Tryptophan actually is the precursor to this soporific neurohormone, which is made from serotonin in the brain's pineal gland. And serotonin is a sleeping potion in its own right. So tryptophan is a double-barrelled natural sedative. Its ability, in ample doses (usually 1 to 5 g, taken 30 to 45 minutes before bedtime), to ease many insomniacs into sleep has been documented in dozens of studies (Schneider-Helmert and Spinweber, 1986). But like melatonin, tryptophan's effect wears off early in the night for some people. As for severe, chronic cases of insomnia, they may take weeks to respond, or paradoxically, relief may come only when they stop taking the tryptophan! For these insomniacs, "interval therapy"—a few days on, a few days off—is often the ticket.

NEUROLOGIC AND DEVELOPMENTAL DISORDERS

Serotonin's involvement in disorders of the mind and brain sometimes runs deep into the neurologic and developmental domains.

Parkinson's Disease

If you've seen the movie "Awakenings," or read the book by Oliver Sacks, you've witnessed the wonder of the wonder drug L-dopa—and the horror. Dramatically awakened by it from a long Parkinsonian slumber, Robert De Niro's character soon awakens too much. He becomes a grotesquely twitching, jerking ball of tics—a man who looks very much like someone in whom dopamine, the neurotransmitter made from L-dopa which slowly vanishes in the course of Parkinson's disease (PD), has gained the upper hand over another major movement-regulating neurotransmitter: serotonin. Indeed, he looks like someone who could benefit from another precursor that, coincidentally, neurologists across the ocean were beginning to use, back in the 1960s, to sedate the erratic muscle jerks—the myoclonus—of a different group of patients: 5-HTP.

Not just the florid symptoms of dopamine excess (which include paranoia and visual hallucinations), but also the sluggishness of dopamine deficiency, the depression that afflicts 50 percent of PD sufferers, and the on/off alternations between these extremes have all been attributed, in part, to a related deficiency, common in PD, of serotonin. Some researchers have taken the obvious clinical leap. Their studies, which have yielded wildly mixed results, suggest that while serotonin boosting sometimes worsens PD by upsetting the delicate balance between dopamine and serotonin even more, at other times it is a godsend. For one lucky patient, a low 100 mg/day dose of 5-HTP, with adjunctive carbidopa (a drug often prescribed to minimize the conversion of 5-HTP to serotonin before it reaches the brain), resolved her severe, untreatable depression and markedly improved her PD for at least two years. Each of three times she was switched to a placebo she promptly relapsed (Klein et al., 1986).

Other Movement Disorders

Low brain serotonin is a common finding in disorders of movement control, and serotonin precursors are a commonly investigated therapy.

Myoclonus has proven the most responsive (Pranzatelli, 1994). Though 5-HTP has sometimes exacerbated this muscle-jerking disorder, more often it has been mildly to markedly helpful, particularly for posthypoxic myoclonus.

There is weaker evidence that 5-HTP may be of modest and very gradual benefit to some people with ataxia. 5-HTP and tryptophan have occasionally been reported to be therapeutic for hyperekplexia and dystonia. And tryptophan may also improve some cases of tardive dyskinesia.

Autism

In a large survey, one biomedical treatment received the most praise from parents of autistic children: megadoses of two nutrients that are required for serotonin synthesis, vitamin B6 and magnesium. Parents' favorable reviews outnumbered bad ones ten to one (Rimland, 1988). The reviews have been just as good in over a dozen clinical trials (Pfeiffer et al., 1995).

A problem with serotonin is the most consistent biochemical abnormality in people with autism, affecting about one in three (McDougle et al., 1993). Oddly enough, the problem is high serotonin; but it's high in the blood, where tryptophan is low (D'Eufemia et al., 1995). This suggests that excessive production of serotonin outside the brain could be promoting a deficiency within the brain. Certainly, the symptoms that bedevil autistic people are consistent with this: compulsiveness, depression, hypersensitivity to stimuli, violent or self-abusive behavior and more. Even their penchant for repetitive movements could be an instinctive attempt at serotonergic self-medication (Jacobs, 1991). Significantly, medications that boost brain serotonin, not lower it, are distinguishing themselves in improving the autist's lot.

Natural SBs have barely been investigated. In one trial, low doses of 5-HTP and L-dopa brought improvement to some very young autistic children and deterioration to others, probably because of the L-dopa (Naruse et al., 1989). In a brief experimental study, a young autistic woman's blood tryptophan level was acutely reduced by nearly 90 percent. Her symptoms flared. When it was boosted above baseline by 27 percent, she improved (McDougle et al., 1993). There is also weak or preliminary evidence that the serotonin-boosting vitamin folic acid and a related SB, tetrahydrobiopterin, may benefit children with autism and a similar condition called fragile X syndrome (Naruse et al., 1989).

Tourette Syndrome

Not only does their bottomless bag of tics and their proneness to obsessive-compulsive, self-injurious and aggressive behavior seem to proclaim that people with Tourette syndrome are victims of too much driven dopamine/not enough sedate serotonin, so does their physiology, right down to their genes (Comings, 1990). Fueling the problem, these studies suggest, may be an excessive conversion of tryptophan to a noxious metabolite called kynurenine, leaving little of the amino acid for the brain. Supplements of tryptophan, 5-HTP, and vitamins B3 and B6, which could allay this quirk, have proven effective in a few unconfirmed reports (Yaryura-Tobias, 1979).

OTHER USES

There is much more to serotonin's potential than this brief guide can hope to convey. Here are a few other conditions that may sometimes respond to a serotonin solution.

SBs are becoming a treatment of choice for premenstrual syndrome. Tryptophan has performed well in two of three clinical trials (Brzezinski,1996). Serotonin-boosting drugs, including tryptophan as an adjunct (Watson and Philips, 1986), are making inroads in the treatment of self-injurious behavior (compulsive self-mutilation, paradoxically to bring relief from mental pain). Serotonin seems to act as a brake on the dopamine-fueled flight from reality of schizophrenia and psychosis. Clinical research suggests these disorders can sometimes respond to natural SBs like tryptophan, 5-HTP and vitamin B3 (Yaryura-Tobias et al., 1977; Wittenborn, 1974).

There are indications that several forms of epilepsy — minor partial seizures, grand mal epilepsy, seizures provoked by external stimuli and (especially) progressive myoclonus epilepsy (PME)—can sometimes be buffered by serotonergic agents, including tryptophan and 5-HTP (Pranzatelli, 1994). (But watch out: 5-HTP has provoked status epilepticus in one patient with PME.) Tryptophan may not only be an antidote for the severe tics caused by Ritalin in children with attention deficit hyperactivity disorder (Chandler et al., 1989), but, like serotonergic drugs, it shows signs of relieving the condition itself (Nemzer et al., 1986).

Serotonergic medications, including tryptophan, are among the best antidotes for the behavioral symptoms of Alzheimer's disease and other forms of senile dementia. But there is also good evidence that serotonin boosting can spark cognitive improvements in a lucky few. In one small trial, for instance, 5-HTP and tyrosine combined (tyrosine boosts dopamine and norepinephrine) restored short-term memory to one demented woman, and much of a demented man's ability to care for himself at home (Meyer et al., 1977).

SEROTONIN BOOSTERS

SBs come in two basic types: selective and nonselective. Selective SBs (SSBs), like Prozac and tryptophan, appear to do little or nothing of significance other than boost serotonin. Nonselective SBs (NSBs), like most MAOIs and 5-HTP (which can boost norepinephrine), do, which can make them more useful for some people with serotonin-related conditions, less useful (or even contraindicated) for others.

Of course, SSBs and NSBs also come in both pharmaceutical and natural varieties. Compared with natural SBs, drugs are pushier: while tryptophan and 5-HTP are converted by the brain to serotonin at its pleasure, serotonin reuptake inhibitors like Prozac and Anafranil aggressively block the reuptake (reabsorption) of serotonin by the neurons that release it, thereby extending its effect, whether the neurons like it or not. This isn't necessarily a bad thing. Sometimes only a bad cop can soften up a stubborn chemical imbalance.

Interestingly, some herbal SBs also are SRIs (serotonin reuptake inhibitors that are not selectively serotonergic) or MAOIs; but their gentle effects suggest they are weaker than their synthetic counterparts or that nature has balanced them internally for greater user-friendliness.

Perhaps you're wondering if a combination of good and bad cops might deliver the best of both worlds. In many studies, tryptophan, combined with serotonergic drugs, has proven superior to either party alone. And three-way "cocktails" of tryptophan, lithium, Anafranil and/or progesterone (also an SB) have saved patients when nothing else could.

Unfortunately, these combinations have sometimes pushed people's serotonergic systems too far, provoking a florid serotonin syndrome marked by confusion, delirium, fever, shivering, sweating and other neurologic, gastrointestinal and cardiac symptoms. In a few cases, this syndrome has escalated to life-threatening, even fatal, shock or hyperpyrexia (extreme fever).

While the serotonin syndrome has put a chill on the casual use of highly serotonergic combinations, some experts feel the risks are small compared with the benefits when administred vigilantly to carefully selected patients (Young, 1991A).

ARE SEROTONIN BOOSTERS FOR YOU?

Obviously, the more symptoms or conditions you have that can respond to SBs, the more likely yours will too. Though seldom used outside research settings, certain lab tests may also be of predictive value.

The first test is a measurement of the ratio in the blood of tryptophan (T) to the other large neutral amino acids (LNAA) that compete with it for passage across the blood-brain barrier. While a normal fasting T/LNAA doesn't rule out central serotonin deficiency, a low ratio all but rules it in and not only suggests SBs will be therapeutic but at which dosage (Moller, 1980).

The second test, which involves a painful spinal tap, measures serotonin's breakdown product, 5-HIAA, in the cerebrospinal fluid (CSF). Low CSF 5-HIAA is the gold standard for estimating low serotonin levels or activity in the brain.

TRYPTOPHAN AND 5-HTP

Only a tiny portion of the gram or two of tryptophan we eat each day finds its way into the brain, where serotonergic neurons convert it to 5-HTP and then serotonin.

Thanks to well-timed supplements of tryptophan or 5-HTP, millions of people have bolstered their brain's usual supply of serotonin, relieving their depression, chronic pain and other conditions, with few or no side effects. But some users have taken a bruising—and not just from the catastrophic eosinophilia-myalgia syndrome (EMS) wrought by tryptophan in 1989.

The Eosinophilia-Myalgia Syndrome

The eosinophilia-myalgia syndrome (EMS) afflicted thousands, killed dozens and lingers in hundreds of victims to this day. It resembles a chronic autoimmune disease, with aching joints and muscles, elevated white blood cells (eosinophils), fever, skin rash and fibrosis (hardening), swollen limbs, weakness and such long-term complications as lung disease (including pulmonary hypertension) and cognitive impairment.

Based on overwhelming evidence, there is a virtual consensus among authorities that the EMS epidemic was due not to tryptophan itself, but to contaminated lots of tryptophan from a major Japansese manufacturer, Showa Denko. Unfortunately, this was not the only time that EMS or EMS-like symptoms occured in users of tryptophan and 5-HTP. Eosinophilia, scleroderma-like lesions and even primary pulmonary hypertension have made rare appearances before and since. In one case a Showa Denko-like impurity was found in the 5-HTP. Some experts now wonder if mild, sporadic contamination has always been a problem with tryptophan and 5-HTP and/or if these nutrients may be inherently toxic.

There are, in fact, several normal products of tryptophan metabolism that, in excess, have been implicated in certain diseases, including AIDS dementia, bladder tumors, cataracts, Parkinson's disease and scleroderma.

Serotonin itself is one such toxic metabolite. Moderate peripheral excesses account for many of the side effects of tryptophan and 5-HTP. Extreme excesses are implicated in something more serious: fibrosis in the skin (scleroderma) and in the right chamber of the heart. While there have been no reports of heart fibrosis in tryptophan and 5-HTP users, sclerodermatous lesions are rare side effects—and common symptoms of EMS.

So the bad news is that tryptophan and 5-HTP may pose inherent dangers. The better news is that, save for the bad Showa Denko lots, in many millions of patient years of use, only a few dozen cases of drastic or life-threatening reactions have been reported. Were the statistics much worse, it is doubtful that tryptophan and 5-HTP would still be available in pharmacies in Canada (tryptophan only) and Europe, through compounding pharmacies and as investigational drugs in the United States, in the mail order catalogs of several American and foreign retailers and in the liquid meal replacements of hospital patients and infants (tryptophan only).

Side Effects

Taken as directed, tryptophan and 5-HTP are far better tolerated than their pharmaceutical alternatives. Apparent side effects of tryptophan (including a few paradoxical ones) include agitation, appetite loss, ataxia, blurred vision, constipation, diarrhea, dizziness, drowsiness, dry mouth, headaches, heartburn, hostility, increased aggressiveness, light-headedness, nausea, sexual disinhibition, stomach pain, tremors and vomiting. Such reactions may be minimized if tryptophan is taken with certain supplements, as described below. Likewise for 5-HTP, whose adverse reactions include aggravation of anxiety, hypomania, mania and some serious skin reactions (dermatitis, scleroderma).

Cautions and Contraindications

While tryptophan can therapeutically lower blood pressure, it may also transiently elevate it. Some authorities recommend caution in using tryptophan if you have liver disease or hypoglycemia. Based on the potential metabolic dangers, one very cautious expert recommends against tryptophan (and possibly 5-HTP) supplementation for children and pregnant women, women on estrogens or oral contraceptives and anyone with chronic bladder irritation, lack of stomach acid, overgrowth of gastrointestinal microorganisms, upper bowel malabsorption or a history of cancer, diabetes or scleroderma-like conditions (Sourkes, 1983). These contraindications may be softened by the following adjunctive strategies.

Minimizing the Dangers of Tryptophan and 5-HTP

The best way to minimize potential side effects of tryptophan and 5-HTP is to take adjunctive supplements. Many of the hazards of tryptophan and 5-HTP are due to shortages of the nutrients needed for their safe metabolism. Tryptophan may be noxious for women on estrogen, for example, because estrogen interferes with vitamin B6, which is a key catalyst in tryptophan metabolism. Though far from an exact science, a reasonable estimate based on available evidence would be: for every 500 mg of tryptophan (and perhaps every 50 mg of 5-HTP), take at least 10 mg of B6, 25 mg of B3, 100 mcg of folic acid, 100 mg of C and 50 IU of vitamin E. Extra methionine or SAM might also help—perhaps 100 mg of methionine per 1000 mg of tryptophan (or 100 mg of 5-HTP). However, high doses may be too stimulating for some people. Adequate chromium intake (discussed below) is also important. Much of this prescription can come from a good diet and a well-endowed multivitamin/mineral supplement. One special concern: Too much vitamin B6 could promote premature conversion of 5-HTP to serotonin before it enters the brain. This is especially likely if carbidopa—a drug commonly prescribed with 5-HTP to block this peripheral conversion—isn't being taken, too. One approach would be to start by taking 5-HTP with no more than a few mg of B6, perhaps at a different time of day, and add more B6 later if it doesn't interfere with the clinical effect.

Time your doses for optimum effect. Tryptophan only crosses the blood-brain barrier (BBB)—that is, it passes from the bloodstream into brain tissue—by hitching a ride on a special transport macromolecule. Several other large, electrically neutral amino acids (LNAA) also ride this bus, and usually they crowd tryptophan out. The exception is when we eat food high in carbohydrates (sugars or starches) and low in protein: the resulting insulin response clears most of the competing LNAA from the blood. If we take tryptophan or 5-HTP long after eating protein or soon after eating carbohydrate on a "protein-free stomach," much more will make it into the brain and much less may wind up in the liver, skin, heart, lungs or other peripheral sites where harmful metabolites could be generated. As discussed below, a negative ionizer could also deter peripheral serotonin production.

If you intend to take tryptophan or 5-HTP long-term, consider having your blood or urine screened for abnormal concentrations of the following undesirable metabolites: kynurenine, quinolinic acid and serotonin.

Combining Tryptophan or 5-HTP with Other SBs

As we've seen, combining tryptophan with powerful serotonergic drugs, including lithium, has sometimes resulted in a dangerous serotonin syndrome. The same risk likely applies to 5-HTP. Could a strong brew of purely natural SBs also provoke the syndrome? It's never been reported, but users should be on guard, nonetheless.

Taking Tryptophan and 5-HTP

Tryptophan's dosage ranges from about 500 mg to a dozen or more grams a day (usually in two to four doses), with 1 to 6 g/day suiting most users. 5-HTP's full dosage range is about 50 to 1200 mg/day; its usual range is 100-600 mg/day. Timing, as discussed above, can greatly influence the required dosage. Less tryptophan or 5-HTP may also be needed if one uses supplements that foster serotonin synthesis: vitamins B3, B6, C and E, biotin, folic acid, methionine and the minerals copper, iron, magnesium, manganese and zinc. Anxiety, and perhaps other adverse reactions, can occur if 5-HTP (and maybe tryptophan) is started at a high dosage. Starting low and building gradually will also reduce the risk of overshooting a therapeutic window. If clinical response fades, it may be necessary to raise or lower the dosage or to boost other "needy neurotransmitters" with tyrosine, phenylalanine or methionine (Baumel, 1995).

DIET

When it comes to diet, serotonin is planted in the eye of not one but two storms of controversy.

The Carbohydrate Confusion

As we've seen, when we eat a high carbohydrate meal or snack, insulin clears the path for more tryptophan to cross the blood-brain barrier. As brain serotonin presumably rises, so does the comfort level of most so-called carbohydrate cravers, no matter whether they've just eaten a plate of whole-wheat pasta or a fistful of jelly beans (Sayegh et al., 1995). But their relief from confusion, depression, OCD, tension or other kinds of malaise is short-lived. Hours later their symptoms may be worse than when they started.

Are these serotonin fixes part of the solution or part of the problem? MIT nutritionist Judith Wurtman favors the former hypothesis. Her prescription for carbohydrate cravers (CCers) is to keep doing what they're doing—only better (Wurtman and Suffes, 1996). Skip the greasy potato chips (the fat may obstruct the serotonin effect) and eat a baked potato; resist sweet-and-sour meatballs (the protein will flood the blood with competing LNAA) and suck a lollipop.

A lollipop! To doctors on the other side of the debate from Wurtman, this is a battle cry. Lollipops and other refined carbohydrates—sugar and white versions of everything brown like wheat and rice—are the stuff of which reactive hypoglycemia (RH) is made. RH results from an insulin overreaction to sweets or other rapidly digested carbohydrates. The excess insulin not only sends tryptophan's competition running, it sends blood sugar reeling. With the plug suddenly pulled on the brain's energy supply, people with RH often lose their cool two to four hours after satisfying their carbohydrate hunger (Baumel, 1995; Taylor and Rachman, 1988). An optional surge of adrenal stress hormones to pull fresh sugar from the liver can add its own panicky coloration to the hypoglycemic attack. One symptom inevitably occurs: the renewed craving for another quick carbohydrate fix.

Doctors are divided about how to diagnose RH. The traditionalists demand that symptoms coincide with an abnormally low blood sugar nadir. Most nutritionally oriented doctors and alternative practitioners use a wider diagnostic net, which is better supported by basic research (Baumel, 1995). Even by traditional criteria, several small studies have found RH in most women with panic disorder, phobias and PMS (for example, Denicoff et al., 1990). And in collaborative investigations from the University of Helsinki and the National Institute on Alcohol Abuse and Alcoholism, a smoking serotonergic gun has also been found.

Since the early 1980s, psychiatrists Marku Linnoila and Matti Virkkunen have been taking the measure of impulsive criminals, men typically with a record from childhood of impulsively violent, explosive or antisocial behavior (often including attempted suicide) and alcoholism, like their fathers before them. Low CSF 5-HIAA—suggesting low brain serotonin—has repeatedly been found in most of these men. And so has carbohydrate craving and reactive hypoglycemia. Linnoila and Virkkunen suspect that in these men a chronic serotonin deficiency upsets a regulatory brain center, leading to RH. And the "hypoglycemia directly lowers [their] threshold for impulsive violent behavior" (Linnoila and Virkkunen, 1992).

Linnoila and Virkkunen see serotonergic medications as the solution. But the hypoglycemia-oriented practitioners mentioned above favor a dietary prescription, not only for liquor-loving hellraisers, but for RH patients with all manner of serotonin-related disorders. And in a few small controlled trials, their diets have delivered the goods (Baumel, 1995; Christensen et al., 1991).

The original RH diet, which is an extremely high protein and fat regime, with just a trace of complex carbohydrates (starchy foods) allowed, is still preferred by some doctors (for example, Newbold, 1975). But some people only feel miserable on it.

In contrast, the late naturopath Paavo Airola advocated an unrefined complex carbohydrate bonanza, with a touch of fruit and a moderate intake of protein and fat. It was Airola's popular approach that was prescribed in the successful clinical studies.

More recently, the dietary focus has shifted from preventing RH to boosting serotonin. Hence, the lollipops and other powerful insulin- and serotonin-boosting refined carbohydrates (Wurtman and Suffes, 1996). But others have prescribed a more temperate, Airola-like regime to boost serotonin (Pollack, 1986).

The happy medium between these extremes, in the opinion of psychiatrist Michael Norden (1995), is the popular "zone diet" of scientist Barry Sears. In it 30 percent of calories come from "good fats," 40 percent from good (unrefined) carbohydrates and 30 percent from protein.

And it's a diet that isn't afraid of cholesterol.

The Cholesterol Connection

Usually, low cholesterol means fewer heart attacks. But there's a problem. In most studies, it also means more depression, more suicide, more fatal accidents and more death by homicide. Indeed, cholesterol lowering—with drugs, diet or both—has usually not only failed to lower mortality, it even doubled it in one major trial (Norden, 1995). There is no relief in the epidemiologic literature, which includes the repeated finding of low cholesterol in a now familiar cast of characters: boys with aggressive conduct disorder and men who have been violent and alcoholic since boyhood (Kaplan et al., 1994).

Is this research trying to tell us something? Many experts think it is (Kaplan et al., 1994; Norden, 1995). Consider the fact that in monkeys extra cholesterol at the table makes for sweeter-tempered apes, with higher levels of 5-HIAA in their CSF. Consider the fact that cholesterol abounds in neuronal membranes where it helps serotonin bind to the receptors that heed its laid-back call.

Many scientists are aghast at the thought that cholesterol could be a benign SB. But others see it as vindication of the biochemical which is the mother of all our steroid hormones and a pillar in the membranes of our cells. Besides, only a tiny fraction of our cholesterol—the blood-bound lot that chooses to plug our arteries—gives the rest a bad name. And perhaps that's a key to the puzzle.

Only the "bad" cholesterol in the bloodstream—the LDL-cholesterol (LDL-C)—plugs arteries. "Good" HDL-cholesterol (HDL-C) in the blood actually lowers the risk of cardiovascular disease. Yet many cholesterol-lowering drugs and diets lower both the good and the bad. In fact, I've noticed a trend for trials of such regimes, but not of regimes where

HDL-C is raised, to be plagued by those symptoms of too little serotonin. Significantly, in at least one human study, higher blood levels of HDL-C has meant higher CSF levels of 5-HIAA (that is, higher serotonin), but no such effect for LDL-C (Engstrom et al., 1995). On the other hand, in the monkey-pacifying study, a high cholesterol diet cut HDL-C in half and nearly doubled CSF 5-HIAA.

Health writer A. S. Gissen (1996) has another theory. Gissen notes that in most cholesterol-lowering trials, patients have been told to replace animal fat with vegetable oil. But there's a problem. Supermarket vegetable oils are unnaturally lacking in polyunsaturated fatty acids (PUFA) of the omega-3 family. Omega-3s, unlike any other PUFA, raise HDL. And in the brain, they're the PUFA of choice for supple neuronal membranes—especially the membranes where neurotransmitters (like serotonin) do their work. Could omega-3 deficiency bear at least some responsibility for the serotonin effect? Well, in cross-national research, low omega-3 intake correlates with up to a tenfold increase in depression. And in one epidemiologic study, people who ate lots of fish, which are rich in omega-3 PUFA, had low serum cholesterol (good and bad combined), but fewer instances, not more, of typical hyposerotonergic markers: violent death (suggestive of a violent life) and suicide. Interestingly, the inland brethren of the study's coastal Finns were not big on fish. For them, low cholesterol did not bring less violent death and suicide.

Some psychiatrists are using omega-3-rich supplements like linseed oil and fish oil to treat serotonin-related disorders (Rudin and Felix, 1987; Norden, 1995). "The most complete cure of seasonal [winter] depression that I've ever seen from a single treatment—and I specialize in treating the condition" is how University of Seattle's Michael Norden describes the response of one of his patients, who was given both EPA (eicosapentanoic acid), an important omega-3 fatty acid found in fish and wild game, and a smaller balancing dose of the important omega-6 PUFA, gamma-linolenic acid (GLA).

An Ideal Diet for Raising Serotonin Safely?

Obviously, there are too many holes in our knowledge to make for an easy one-size-fits-all prescription for a nutritious serotonin-boosting diet. But based on the best current evidence, here are some suggestions.

First comes fat. Putting the cholesterol issue aside for now, a diet in which all or most fat is "good fat" is consistent both with good health and serotonin boosting. Good fat means fat (usually oil) that is as fresh and unrefined as possible and reasonably consistent in make-up with the climate you live in. The cooler the climate, the higher the need for unsaturated fatty acids, especially omega-3s, which are well-represented (in roughly descending order of omega-3 content) in cold water fish and seafood, flax seeds (and linseed oil), wild game, walnuts, hazelnuts, pumpkin seeds, beans, whole wheat and dark green vegetables.

As for cholesterol, we make the stuff ourselves, so avoiding it—as vegans, who are probably the healthiest people on the planet, do—shouldn't usually be a problem. But some people may simply not be able to make as much cholesterol as they need for adequate serotonergic function. For them, eating wholesome foods that are high in cholesterol (eggs, seafood, organ meats—brains are the biggest cholesterol fix on earth) could (gulp) be safe and beneficial, especially if antioxidants like vitamins C and E are taken to lower the atherosclerotic risk and if a doctor monitors the ratio of good (HDL) to bad (LDL) cholesterol in their blood.

Any serotonin-friendly diet will have to include at least some carbohydrates. The question is, which kind? I side with those who would keep refined carbohydrates to a minimum. Only nature's unrefined packages reliably provide enough fiber, chromium and other nutrients required for their smooth and safe handling. Refined carbohydrates may provoke a faster, flashier blood sugar > insulin > serotonin response, but that surge of insulin seems to promote degenerative diseases (Norden, 1995), and the quick-fix effect reeks of drug dependency, with its recurring binge/crash cycles.

Wouldn't wholesome unrefined carbohydrates accomplish the same serotonergic end more gently, moderately and healthfully?

The discussion of carbohydrate food choices would be incomplete without mentioning the glycemic index (GI). Developed primarily as a guide for diabetics, the GI is a measure of the rise in blood sugar that follows the ingestion of carbohydrate-rich foods. Surprisingly, wholesome carbohydrate foods sometimes have GIs higher than their junky counterparts. Whole grain bread, for instance, has a higher GI than table sugar! But the GI only measures the quantity, not the quality of the blood sugar rise and fall. A bowl of jelly beans could send blood sugar soaring for 90 minutes, then plummeting, while a bowl of bulgur could send it up a gentle slope for the entire three-hour GI period. The bulgur might yield a higher GI than the jelly beans, but the jelly beans would have provoked reactive hypoglycemia in some people, and the bulgur would not.

As we've seen, protein, which is where amino acids come from, is no friend to serotonin boosting. Fortunately, most of us are already eating about twice as much protein as nutritionists think we need. What's more, most people's carbohydrate cravings only occur at certain times of day, nightime being the prime time. This, therefore, would be the time to ease up on the protein. During the day, bright light exposure may indirectly boost serotonin (see below), allowing us to meet our protein needs without feeling a serotonin pinch. The custom of having your supper at breakfast or lunchtime and your high-carbohydrate breakfast at suppertime could be a recipe for high brain serotonin all day long.

VITAMIN B3 (NIACIN, NIACINAMIDE) AND VITAMIN B6 (PYRIDOXINE)

Vitamin B3 is one vitamin we can actually make ourselves, but only at the cost of another essential nutrient, tryptophan. Indeed, being converted to B3 is tryptophan's usual fate, especially when we're under stress.

Stress could therefore lead to the distress of serotonin deficiency. And, indeed, signs of a mass migration of tryptophan down the pathway to NAD (the active coenzyme form of B3) and of central hyposerotonergia are common among stressed-out psychiatric patients (Hoes, 1989). They also are showing up in people under immunologic stress—people with chronic infectious illnesses like AIDS and chronic fatigue syndrome—which implicates serotonin deficiency in the neuropsychiatric symptoms of these conditions. Ironically, much of this diverted tryptophan never even makes it to NAD. Harmful intermediate metabolites accumulate, instead, apparently due to a lack of vitamin B6, which is required to complete the conversion. With high blood levels of B3 and NAD being the liver's signal to ease up on making them, chronic stress can easily become a profound tryptophan drain.

Supplements of B3 (or NAD) and B6 could plug this drain. It doesn't hurt that these vitamins also help neurons make serotonin. Orthomolecular psychiatrists, who specialize in treating mental disease nutritionally, have long prescribed megadoses of B3 and B6 for the serotonin-related (and other) ills of their patients (for example, Newbold, 1975; Slagle, 1987). Their mostly anecdotal successes have been supported by some, but not all, controlled research (for example, Wittenborn, 1974; Bernstein, 1990; Pfeiffer et al., 1995).

B3 and B6 appear safe and well-tolerated at the moderate dosages required to enhance the safety and efficacy of tryptophan. Slightly higher dosages (up to 500 mg of B3 and 100-200 mg of B6) can be therapeutic in their own right, with little or no risk. But as megadoses climb toward grams a day, the risk of adverse effects, such as liver damage from niacin and nerve damage from B6, and the need to be mindful of medical contraindications and other considerations (Baumel, 1995) make knowledgeable medical supervision advisable, if not essential. However, just as B3 and B6 reduce tryptophan's hazards, a high potency multivitamin and mineral supplement makes B3, B6 and indeed any other nutrient safer, too.

Some people have trouble converting pyridoxine, niacin or niacinamide to their activated coenzyme forms: pyridoxal-5-phosphate and NAD. These coenzymes are available as supplements and should be effective at much lower doses than B3 or B6.

SAM AND METHIONINE

In Italy SAM (s-adenosylmethionine [ademetionine, Gumbaral]) is one of the most commonly prescribed antidepressants. With numerous controlled clinical trials indicating that SAM is at least as effective as antidepressant drugs, but far better tolerated (Bressa, 1994), SAM is generating excitement on this side of the Atlantic, too (Fava et al., 1995).

A natural product of the essential amino acid methionine, SAM in the brain boosts serotonin (Young, 1991B) and perhaps norepinephrine and dopamine, too. In preliminary trials, SAM has appeared helpful for dementia, fibromyalgia, residual (adult) attention deficit hyperactivity disorder and migraine.

While SAM itself is very expensive (roughly $5 to $15 a day), methionine could be an affordable and effective substitute. Methionine actually crosses the blood-brain barrier more readily than SAM (Braverman et al., 1997). Anecdotally, it has been effective both for depression and for an obsessive-compulsive subgroup of schizoaffective people.

SAM (and probably methionine) seems to be a stimulating nonselective SB, capable of provoking anxiety, restlessness and (mostly in bipolar users) mania or hypomania. But generally it is well-tolerated. In a huge and successful clinical trial of SAM for osteoarthritis, just 5 percent of more than 20,000 patients quit because of side effects (Berger and Nowak, 1987). SAM's dosage is usually 600 to 1600 mg/day; methionine's is 1-2 g. Both should be balanced with a generous intake of vitamins B6 and C, folic acid, calcium and magnesium.

FOLIC ACID

The B vitamin folic acid (also known as folate) helps the brain synthesize dopamine, norepinephrine, SAM, serotonin and a compound named tetrahydrobiopterin, which seems to stimulate the release of serotonin and other neurotransmitters. Deficiencies of folic acid are endemic among alcoholics, depressives, epileptics, people with chronic fatigue syndrome and neuropsychiatric patients in general. In most controlled studies, treating the deficiency has relieved psychiatric symptoms, and high folate levels (naturally or from supplements) have promoted response to lithium or antidepressant drugs and reduced relapse among recovered bipolars and depressives. In other trials, megadoses of folate's more active metabolite, methylfolate, have been an acute antidepressant and have benefited folate-deficient schizophrenics, too (Young, 1991B).

Therapeutic doses of folate and methylfolate usually range from a few milligrams up to 80 mg/day. One psychiatrist's patients tend to feel stimulated, sedated or "just rotten" on megadoses of folate (Newbold, 1975). Dose-dependent side effects include anxiety, hyperactivity, insomnia, irritabilty and possibly a lowered seizure threshold. Sometimes responders must lower the dosage after a while to maintain benefits.

LITHIUM

A commonplace natural element like sodium and potassium, lithium in megadoses is one of psychiatry's most versatile "drugs" (Lenox and Manji, 1995). It is a mood stabilizer for bipolar disorder, a heavy-hitting adjunct for acute depression and a venerable maintenance therapy, a pacifier for violent children and adults, an admittedly elusive would-be antidote for alcoholism, a top-notch treatment for cluster headache and a promising treatment for PMS and adjunctively OCD. If this sounds like the profile of a serotonin booster, it's because lithium is.

Usually prescribed in near-toxic supermegadoses, lithium has sometimes proven effective at much lower, better-tolerated doses (as little as 150 to 300 mg/day), especially when used adjunctively.

MAGNESIUM

A catalyst for serotonin synthesis (among its innumerable other activities), the mineral magnesium may be medicine for several hyposerotonergic conditions. Combined with vitamin B6, it allays autism (Rimland, 1988; Pfeiffer et al., 1995). In some trials, injections have lifted mood and relieved aches and pains, lethargy and weakness, in people with depression or chronic fatigue syndrome (Baumel, 1995). It can be a potent mood stabilizer for bipolar disorder (Chouinard et al., 1990). And there is evidence that it sometimes relieves anxiety, attention deficit hyperactivity disorder, insomnia and PMS.

With increasing dosage (the usual range is from 400-1200 mg/day; much less for organic chelates), magnesium becomes less energizing and more tranquilizing or even (in excess) depressing.

CHROMIUM

Chromium is a trace mineral that vanishes without a trace when carbohydrates are refined. Yet the body needs chromium to process those carbohydrates: without it, insulin can't ferry sugar from the blood into the tissues. Possibly, chromium deficiency also impairs insulin's ability to do the same for tryptophan's LNAA competitors. Such an impairment might explain why obese carbohydrate cravers—who tend to be both insulin resistant and chromium deficient— appear to have LNAA that linger long in the bloodstream, with carbohydrates failing to produce the expected rise in their T/LNAA ratio (Caballero et al., 1988). This could account for many a return trip to the cookie jar in vain pursuit of a serotonin fix. Chromium supplements, which have at least helped rats make fewer trips to the cookie jar, might also help humans get the most serotonergic punch for the least carbohydrate lunch.

ST. JOHN'S WORT (HYPERICUM)

There are many herbs with age-old reputations as psychiatric cure-alls, banishers of demons, wards against evil—the whole hyperbolic bit. But none delivers the scientific goods like St. John's Wort (SJW). In roughly two dozen controlled clinical trials involving nearly 2000 mostly mildly to moderately depressed patients, SJW has usually proven markedly superior to placebo, equal to low doses of antidepressant drugs and virtually free of side effects (Linde et al., 1996). In Germany, medical doctors prescribe SJW far more often than Prozac. On the Internet, where SJW is hot, some users prefer it to SSRIs.

SJW is a mild MAOI—too mild, researchers suspect, to account for its benefits. The credit may belong to another apparent effect of SJW: serotonin reuptake inhibition (Perovic and Muller, 1995). Certainly the herb's range of clinical benefits do not contradict this. SJW may equal bright light for winter depression (Martinez et al., 1994); it is licensed in Germany for treating anxiety, depression and sleep disorders; it's traditionally indicated for pain (sciatica, menstrual cramps, headache); and, of course, it keeps the demons away—the kind, perhaps, that we recognize today as disorders of impulse control, obsession and compulsion.

The usual dosage of SJW is 300 mg, taken three times a day, of a powdered extract standardized to contain 0.3 percent hypericin. On Internet newsgroups, some users report having headaches, high blood pressure or other reactions that suggest SJW's MAOI effect may sometimes be strong enough to necessitate avoiding foods, beverages and medications that interact in this way with MAOI drugs.

GINKGO BILOBA

Best known and documented as a treatment for mental decline and dementia, the herb ginkgo biloba includes among its many physiological effects some complex connections with serotonin (White et al., 1996). Its apparent MAOI effect should preserve the neurotransmitter; its stimulating effect on serotonergic neuron autoreceptors should dampen serotonergic activity. Together, research suggests, these effects could preserve serotonin in the face of chronic stress and aging. In keeping with this, one of ginkgo's licensed indications in Germany is for "emotional instability with anxiety" (Kleijnen and Klipschild, 1992). And a compound in ginkgo—bilobalide—is patented as a treatment for anxiety and depression (White et al., 1996).

At a typical dosage of 40 or 60 mg, taken three times a day, ginkgo (standardized to contain 24 percent glycosides and, sometimes, 6 percent terpenes) has been remarkably safe and well-tolerated in millions of patient years of usage (Kleijnen and Klipschild, 1992).

HORMONES

Long before scientists knew about neurotransmitters, there were hormones to explain people's behavior. Today, it is becoming increasingly apparent that hormones and neurotransmitters are a highly intimate and interactive family. And when it comes to serotonin, the sex hormones are its most conspicuous bedfellows.

Testosterone antagonizes serotonin; it prefers dynamic dopamine. Estrogen has mixed, hard-to-read feelings, though its affection for sanguine norepinephrine and its antagonism to serotonin-boosting vitamin B6 are clear. Progesterone is one of the best friends serotonin ever had, an SRI and an inhibitor of serotonin breakdown all in one (Chouinard et al., 1987).

All these hormones have been used clinically in ways suggestive of their neurotransmitter effects: estrogen to lift mood and, combined with progesterone, stabilize bipolar mood swings (Chouinard et al., 1987); progesterone to tame sex offenders and other violent criminals and (controversially) PMS; testosterone to put a tiger in the tank of both men and women (Newbold, 1975).

Too much of any one hormone can be as disturbing as too little (Baumel, 1995). High estrogen levels, for example, promote OCD in some women (Weiss et al., 1995). A careful balance of all sex hormones—preferably from well-tolerated natural sources such as phytoestrogen-rich foods (soybeans, flax seeds), natural micronized progesterone or the steroid hormone precursors DHEA and pregnenolone—seems to be the prescription with the most promise.

ACUPUNCTURE

Acupuncture owes its prowess as a pain reliever and mood enhancer not just to its famous endorphin effect, but perhaps even more fundamentally to its lesser known serotonergic effect (Han, 1986). Indeed, stimulating certain acupuncture points boosts both the release of serotonin in the brain and its synthesis. No wonder acupuncture is traditionally indicated for so many serotonin-related conditions. Among those for which modern research lends some support are addictions, depression, headache, insomnia and pain.

EXERCISE

Like a high carbohydrate meal, vigorous exercise clears a path for tryptophan into the brain (Conlay et al., 1989). Indeed, grueling exercise can be so serotonergic, many experts blame this for the "central fatigue" that haunts endurance athletes. Thankfully, moderate exercise boosts serotonin moderately. As for the chronic effect of exercise on serotonin, it's complex and hard to interpret, but the rainbow of psychotherapeutic benefits suggests a benign serotonergic "training effect" is at work.

Foremost among these benefits is exercise's well-established antagonism—on a par with psychotherapy and drugs—to depression: mild, moderate and sometimes even severe (Baumel, 1995). Exercise also reduces tension and anxiety and promotes calm, clearheadedness, poise, self-confidence, superior stress tolerance, vigor, well-being—and a good night's sleep. It may lessen aggressiveness, binge eating, hostility and dysfunctional behavior in general.

Most studies have assessed the psychotherapeutic effects of aerobic exercise: nonexhausting activity that gets your heart beating fast for at least 20 or 30 minutes three times a week. But some studies suggest nonaerobic exercise—weight training, t'ai chi, yoga— can be just as effective. There is even intriguing animal evidence that simple repetitive movements like chewing and licking activate serotonergic neurons (Jacobs, 1991; Norden, 1995). Perhaps this is the basis for knitter's calm, gum chewer's cool and the famous rocking-chair contentment syndrome.

BRIGHT LIGHT THERAPY

People with the fall/winter depression form of seasonal affective disorder (SAD) are as keen a group of carbohydrate cravers as you're ever likely to find. And the most consistently effective medications for their condition are shaping up to be selective serotonin boosters, including tryptophan (Tam et al., 1995). But so is a stiff daily dose of very bright light—unless you cut off the responder's supply of dietary tryptophan (Lam et al., 1996).

For researchers, these and other clues hint strongly at a major role for serotonin deficiency in winter depression, with bright light preserving serotonin from the greedy hand of darkness.

Darkness signals our "third eye," the pineal gland, to convert serotonin into melatonin. Bright light tells it to stop. People who don't get enough bright light may therefore get overloaded with melatonin and deficient in serotonin. High daytime melatonin levels have indeed been documented in people with winter depression, a condition strongly associated with bright light deprivation due to short, cold winter days. The same may prove true for a subgroup of people whose serotonin-related conditions flare up in winter—people with bulimia, OCD (Jenike, 1997), panic disorder, PMS and recurrent brief depressions. But could it also apply to people who shun bright light any time of year? The fact that SAD-like symptoms afflict light-shy San Diegans in the summer certainly suggests it does (Espiritu et al., 1994).

Bright light is by no means a selective booster or preserver of serotonin. Its predominant effect is to stimulate—enough, in high doses, to induce agitation, anxiety, headaches, insomnia, hypomania and mania. This may contraindicate it for some excitable serotonin-shy individuals and recommend it for others. Clinical studies suggest the latter may include people with depression, including the depressive phase of bipolar disorder (use with caution), bulimia and Parkinson's disease.

Bright light therapy can entail sitting near a powerful commercial light box for 30 minutes to two hours a day. But the great light box in the sky should be at least as effective, and pointing ordinary household lamps at a light surface, like a book or a light tabletop so the bright reflected light floods your field of vision, should also do. For safety's sake, the light should be bright, not blinding.

Bright light strongly influences daily biorhythms. People who stay up late and/or oversleep in the morning are likely to benefit most from bright light as early in the day as possible. Those who get tired early and/or wake up early usually benefit from bright light closer to bedtime (Baumel, 1995).

NEGATIVE AIR IONS

In some places, ill winds really do blow. The foehn in Europe, the sharav in Israel, the Santa Ana in California—these and other winds like them stir up symptoms in sensitive individuals that have serotonin deficiency written all over them:

aches and pains, accidents, anxiety, confusion, depression, lethargy, panic attacks, restlessness, sleeplessness, suicide, tension and violent and impulsive antisocial acts (Soyka and Edmunds, 1977).

These winds, it turns out, are laden with masses of positively charged particles or ions, which, at least in weather-sensitive people, cause a nasty build-up of serotonin outside the brain and possibly (the research is inconsistent) a resultant shortage within (Norden, 1995).

Nature's antidote is negative air ions. Not only do these neutralize the positive ion effect, dozens of studies show they tend to make ordinary people feel weller than well—more alert, refreshed and relaxed. The fact that negative air ions reduce excessive peripheral serotonin and seem (again the research is murky) to boost serotonin centrally (in the brain) could also account for preliminary findings that they can rapidly calm manic patients (Misiaszek et al., 1986) and uplift SAD ones (Terman and Terman, 1995).

It is unknown how many people with serotonin-related disorders could secretly be suffering from ill winds or other sources of positive/negative air ion imbalances, such as approaching thunderstorms or warm weather fronts, centrally heated or air-conditioned buildings with poor ventilation, combustion byproducts (cigarette smoke, automobile exhaust) and strong electromagnetic fields. One can't help but think of autistic people, roughly 30 percent of whom are up to their ears in blood serotonin.

Portable electronic negative ionizers are the treatment of choice for this condition. In a recent study, an unusually high-density ionizer equaled bright light therapy for winter depression, but a low-density ionizer didn't (Terman and Terman, 1995). This suggests that the low-density ionizers used in most prior studies—and often found wanting—may be too weak for many people (Norden, 1995).

As of this writing, you won't find 5-HTP, SAM or tryptophan in stores, and you'll have a hard time finding NAD or pyridoxal-5-phosphate, but they are legally available from several other sources. Here are a few (the prescription suppliers are generally much cheaper):

• BIOS Biochemicals (520-326-2385; www.biochemicals. com) sells pyridoxal-5-phosphate and tryptophan without a prescription.
• Medical Center Pharmacy (800-723-7455) is a compounding pharmacy that sells carbidopa, 5-HTP and tryptophan by prescription.
• 5-HTP can be had without prescription from a rapidly growing number of sellers, including Life Link (805-473-1389; www.lifelinknet.com) and Cosmic Sales and Marketing (800-359-9896; www.cris.com/~nubrain); the latter also sells NAD. Some suppliers (for example, Life Enhancement Products (800-543-3873; www.life-enhancement.com) sell a nonsynthetic, plant-derived 5-HTP, alone or with pyridoxal phosphate and a touch of St. John's Wort.
• International Antiaging Systems (011-44-541-514-144; www.worldhealth.net/ias/) sells 5-HTP, SAM and tryptophan.
• Tryptophan is available in Canadian pharmacies by prescription.
• I have not been able to find any suppliers of methylfolate or tetrahydrobiopterin.
• The IonAir Company of Fort Lauderdale (800-478-7324, www.breathe.com) manufactures and sells high density ionizers.

REFERENCES

Due to space constraints, I have had to keep references to a bare minimum. Most of those not included here can be found with minimal effort in the primary medical literature or in the literature on natural/alternative medicine.

Baumel, Syd. 1995. Dealing with Depression Naturally (New Canaan, Conn.: Keats Publishing).

Berger, R., and H. Nowak. Nov. 20, 1987. "A new medical approach to the treatment of osteoarthritis: report of an open phase IV study with ademetionine (Gumbaral)," Am. J. Med. 83: 84-88.

Bernstein, A. L. 1990. "Vitamin B6 in clinical neurology," Ann. N.Y.Acad. Sci. 585: 250-60s.

Blier, P., and R. Bergeron. March 1996. "Sequential administration of augmentation strategies in treatment-resistant obsessive-compulsive disorder: preliminary findings," Inter. Clinics in Psychopharm. (Berlin) 11: 37-44.

Bowen, D. J. et al. April 1991. "Tryptophan and high-carbohydrate diets as adjuncts to smoking cessation therapy," J. Behav. Med. 14: 97-110.

Braverman, Eric. R., et al. 1997. The Healing Nutrients Within: Facts, Findings and New Research on Amino Acids, rev. ed. (New Canaan, Conn.: Keats Publishing).

Bressa, G. M. 1994. "S-adenosyl-l-methionine (SAMe) as antidepressant: meta-analysis of clinical studies," Acta Neurologica Scandinavica 54 (Suppl.): 7-14.

Brzezinski, A. Feb. 17, 1996. "Serotonin and premenstrual dysphoric disorder," Lancet 347:470-71.

Buydens-Branchey, L., et al. March 1989. "Age of alcoholism onset. II. Relationship to susceptibility to serotonin precursor availability," Arch. Gen. Psychiatry 46: 231-36.

Caballero, B., et al. July 1988. "Plasma amino acids and insulin levels in obesity: Response to carbohydrate intake and tryptophan supplements," Metabolism 37: 672-76.

Cangiano, C., et al. Nov. 1992. "Eating behavior and adherence to dietary prescriptions in obese adult subjects treated with 5-hydroxytryptophan," Am. J. Clin. Nutr. 56: 863-67.

Chouinard, G., et al. June 1987. "Estrogen-progesterone combination: another mood stabilizer?" Am. J. Psychiatry 144: 826.

_____ et al. 1990. "A pilot study of magnesium aspartate hydrochloride (magnesiocard) as a mood stabilizer for rapid cycling bipolar affective disorder patients," Prog. Neuro-Psychopharm. & Biol. Psychiatry 14(2): 171-80.

Christensen, L., et al. April 1, 1991. "Dietary alteration of somatic symptoms and regional brain electrical activity," Biol. Psychiatry 29: 679-82.

Clavel, F., et al. Nov. 30, 1985. "Helping people to stop smoking: Randomised comparison of groups being treated with acupuncture and nicotine gum with a control group," Brit. Med. J. 291:1538-39.

Cleare, A. J., and A. J. Bond. March 1995. "The effect of tryptophan depletion and enhancement on subjective and behavioural aggression in normal male subjects," Psychopharmacology (Berlin) 118: 72-81.

Cole, W., and Y. D. LaPierre. Nov. 1986. "The use of tryptophan in normal-weight bulimia," Can. J. Psychiatry 31: 755-56.

Comings, D. E. Aug. 1990. "Blood serotonin and tryptophan in Tourette syndrome," Am. J. Med. Genet. 36: 418-30.

Conlay, L. A., et al. 1989. "Effects of running the Boston Marathon on plasma concentrations of large neutral amino acids," J. Neur. Transmission 76: 65-71.

Denicoff, K. D., et al. Apr. 1990. "Glucose tolerance testing in women with premenstrual syndrome," Am. J. Psychiatry147: 477-80.

D'Eufemia, P, et al. 1995. "Low serum tryptophan to large neutral amino acids ratio in idiopathic infantile autism," Biomed-Pharmacother 49(6): 288-92.

Engstrom, G., et al. Fall 1995. "Serum lipids in suicide attempters," Suicide & Life Threatening Behav. 25: 393-400.

Espiritu, R. C., et al. 1994. "Low illumination experienced by San Diego adults: Association with atypical depressive symptoms," Biol. Psychiatry 35: 398-402.

Fava, M., et al. Apr. 28, 1995. "Rapidity of onset of the antidepressant effect of parenteral S-adenosyl-L-methionine," Psychiatry Res. 56: 295-97.

Gissen, A. S. Jan./Feb. 1996. "Heart disease & depression: The DHA link," Nutr. News 9 (9): 1-4.

Han, J. S. 1986. "Electroacupuncture: An alternative to antidepressants for treating affective diseases?" Inter. J. Neuroscience 29: 79-92.

Hoes, M. J. A. J. M. 1989. "Kynurenines and the affective disorders," in Trevor W. Stone, ed., Quinolinic Acid and the Kynurenines (Boca Raton, Fla.: CRC Press), pp. 229-39.

Jacobs, B. L. Dec. 1991. "Serotonin and behavior: Emphasis on motor control," J. Clin. Psychiatry 52 (Suppl.): 17-23.

Jenike, Michael A., M.D., personal communication, Feb. 1997.

Kahn, R. S., et al. Jan. 1987. "Effect of a serotonin precursor and uptake inhibitor in anxiety disorders; a double-blind comparison of 5-hydroxytryptophan, clomipramine and placebo," Inter. Clin. Psychopharmacol. 2: 33-45.

Kaplan, J. R., et al. 1994. "Demonstration of an association among dietary cholesterol, central serotonergic activity, and social behavior in monkeys," Psychosomatic Med. 56: 479-84.

Kleijnen, J., and P. Knipschild. Nov. 7, 1992. "Ginkgo biloba," Lancet 340: 1136-39.

Klein, P., et al. 1986. "Consequences of chronic 5-hydroxy-tryptophan in Parkinsonian instability of gait and balance and in other neurological disorders," Adv. Neurol. 45: 603-04.

Krahn, D., and J. Mitchell. Sept. 1985. "Use of L-tryptophan in treating bulimia," Am. J. Psychiatry 142: 1130.

Kramer, Peter. 1993. Listening to Prozac (New York: Penguin).

Lam, R. W., et al. Jan. 1996. "Effects of rapid tryptophan depletion in patients with seasonal affective disorder in remission after light therapy," Arch. Gen. Psychiatry 53: 41-44.

Lenox, R. H., and H. K. Manji. 1995. "Lithium," in Alan F. Schatzberg and Charles B. Nemeroff, eds., The American Psychiatric Textbook of Psychopharmacology (Washington, D.C.: American Psychiatric Press, Inc.), pp. 303-49.

Linde, K., et al. Aug. 3, 1996. "St. John's wort for depression: An overview and meta-analysis of randomised clinical trials," Brit. Med. J. 313: 253-58.

Linnoila, V. M., and M. Virkkunen. Oct. 1992. "Aggression, suicidality, and serotonin," J. Clin. Psychiatry 53 (Suppl.): 46-51.

Lion, J. R. 1995. "Aggression," in Harold I. Kaplan and Benjamin J. Sadock, eds., Comprehensive Textbook of Psychiatry, vol. 1 (Baltimore, Md.: Williams & Wilkins)., pp. 310-17.

McDougle, C. J., et al. 1993. "Acute tryptophan depletion in autistic disorder: a controlled case study," Biol. Psychiatry 33: 547-50.

Martinez, B., et al. Oct. 1994. "Hypericum in the treatment of seasonal affective disorders," J. Ger. Psychiatry & Neurol. 7 (Suppl. 1): S29-33.

Meyer, J. S., et al. July 1977. "Neurotransmitter precursor amino acids in the treatment of multiinfarct dementia and Alzheimer's disease," J. Am. Ger. Soc. 25: 89-98.

Misiaszek, J., et al. Jan. 1986. "The calming effect of negative air ions on manic patients," Biol. Psychiatry 22: 107-10.

Moller, S. E., et al. Mar. 1980. "Relationship between plasma ratio of tryptophan to competing amino acids and the response to L-tryptophan," J. Affect. Disorders 2: 47-59.

Morand, C., et al. 1983. "Clinical Response of aggressive schizophrenics to oral tryptophan," Biol. Psychiatry 18 (5): 575-77.

Müller-Oerlinghausen, B., et al. 1992. "The effect of long-term lithium treatment on the mortality of patients with manic-depressive and schizoaffective illness," Acta Psychiatrica Scandinavica 86: 218-22.

Naruse, H., et al. Mar. 1989. "Metabolic changes in aromatic amino acids and monoamines in infantile autism and development of new treatment related to the finding," No To Hattatsu 21: 181-89.

Nemzer, E. D., et al. July 1986. "Amino acid supplementation as therapy for attention deficit disorder," J. Am. Acad. Child Psychiatry 25: 509-13.

Newbold, H. L. 1975. Mega-Nutrients for Your Nerves (New York: Berkley Books).

Norden, Michael J. 1995. Beyond Prozac: Brain-Toxic Lifestyles, Natural Antidotes & New Generation Antidepressants (New York: HarperCollins).

Papaioannou, R., and C. C. Pfeiffer. 1986. "Pure water for drinking," J. Orthomol. Med. 1 (3): 184-98.

Perovic, S., and M. E. G. Muller. 1995. "Pharmacological profile of hypericum extract. Effect of serotonin uptake by postsynaptic receptors," Arzneim Forsch 45: 1145-48.

Pfeiffer, S. I., et al., Oct. 1995. "Efficacy of vitamin B6 and magnesium in the treatment of autism: A methodology review and summary of outcomes," J. Autism & Devel. Disorders 25: 481-93.

Poldinger, W., et al. 1991. "A functional-dimensional approach to depression: Serotonin deficiency as a target symptom in a comparison of 5-hydroxytryptophan and fluvoxamine," Psychopathology 24: 53-81.

Pollack, Robert, et al. 1986. The Pain-Free Tryptophan Diet (New York: Warner Books).

Pranzatelli, M. R. June 1994. "Serotonin and human myoclonus," Arch. Neurology 51: 605-17.

Puttini, P. S., and I. Caruso. Apr. 1992. "Primary fibromyalgia syndrome and 5-hydroxy-L-tryptophan: A 90-day open study," J. Inter. Med. Res. 20: 182-89.

Rimland, B. 1988. "Controversies in the treatment of autistic children: Vitamin and drug therapy," J. Child Neurol. 3 (Suppl.): S68-72.

Rudin, Donald O., and Clare Felix. 1987. The Omega-3 Phenomenon: The Nutrition Breakthrough of the '80s (New York: Rawson Associates).

Sachs, G. S. Dec. 1989. "Adjuncts and alternatives to lithium therapy for bipolar affective disorder," J. Clin. Psychiatry 50 (Suppl.): 31-39.

Sayegh, R., et al. Oct. 1995. "The effect of a carbohydrate-rich beverage on mood, appetite, and cognitive function in women with premenstrual syndrome," Ob. & Gyn. 86: 520-28.

Schneider-Helmert, D., and C. L. Spinweber. 1986. "Evaluation of L-tryptophan for treatment of insomnia: A review," Psychopharmacology (Berlin) 89 (1): 1-7.

Slagle, Priscilla. 1987. The Way Up from Down (New York: Random House).

Sourkes, T. L. 1983. "Toxicology of serotonin precursors," Adv. in Biol. Psychiatry 10: 160-75.

Soyka, Fred, and Alan Edmunds. 1977. The Ion Effect (Toronto: Lester and Orpen).

Strain, G. W., and B. Zumoff. 1985. "L-tryptophan does not increase weight loss in carbohydrate-craving obese subjects," Inter. J. Obesity 9 (6): 375-80.

Tam, E. M., et al. Oct. 1995. "Treatment of seasonal affective disorder: A review," Can. J. Psychiatry 40: 457-66.

Taylor, L. A., and S. J. Rachman. 1988. "The effects of blood sugar level changes on cognitive function, affective state, and somatic symptoms," J. Behav. Med. 11 (3): 279-91.

Terman, M., and J. S. Terman. 1995. "Treatment of seasonal affective disorder with a high-output negative ionizer," J. Alt. & Compl. Med. 1: 87-92.

van Hiele, L. J. 1980. "L-5-hydroxytryptophan in depression: The first substitution therapy in psychiatry?" Neuropsychobiol. 6 (4): 230-40.

van Praag, H. M. 1981. "Management of depression with serotonin precursors," Biol. Psychiatry16 (3): 291-310.

Watson, A. J. S., and K. Philips. 1986. "Serotonergic treatment of screaming and banging in dementia," Lancet 337 (ii): 1464-65.

Weiss, M., et al. May 1995. "The influence of gonadal hormones on periodicity of obsessive-compulsive disorder," Can. J. Psychiatry 40: 205-7.

Weltzin, T. E., et al. Nov. 1995. "Acute tryptophan depletion and increased food intake and irritability in bulimia nervosa," Am. J. Psychiatry 152: 1668-71.

White, H. L., et al. 1996. "Extracts of ginkgo biloba leaves inhibit monoamine oxidase," Life Sci. 58 (16): 1315-21.

Wittenborn, J. R. 1974. "A search for responders to niacin supplementation," Arch. Gen. Psychiatry 31: 547-52.

Wurtman, Judith, and Susan Suffes. 1996. The Serotonin Solution (New York: Fawcett).

Yaryura-Tobias, J. A., et al. 1977. "Tryptophan and perceptual schizophrenias," Orthomol. Psychiatry 6 (2): 1-2.

_____ and H. N. Bhagavan. Nov. 1977. "L-tryptophan in obsessive-compulsive disorders," Am. J. Psychiatry134: 1298-99.

_____. Jan. 1979. "Gilles de la Tourette syndrome. Interactions with other neuropsychiatric disorders," Acta Psychiatrica Scandinavica 59: 9-16.

Young, S. N. Dec. 1991A. "Use of tryptophan in combination with other antidepressant treatments: A review," J. Psychiatry & Neurosci. 16: 241-46.

_____. July 1991B. "The 1989 Borden Award Lecture. Some effects of dietary components (amino acids, carbohydrate, folic acid) on brain serotonin synthesis, mood, and behavior," Can. J. Physiol. & Pharmacol. 69: 893-903.

Ordering Your Free Keats Publishing Catalog is Fast and Easy!

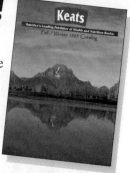

Enjoy a wealth of health-saving information and an opportunity to expand your knowledge of alternative and complementary medicines. Choose from an array of titles spanning the areas of herbal medicine, vitamin supplementation, Oriental medicines, women's health, special diets, homeopathy, acupuncture and much more! Simply complete and mail us the coupon below and receive the complete Keats Publishing catalog free!

OR FOR FASTER ORDERING...

☞ Call our toll-free number **1-800-858-7014** extension **10**

☞ Sample our complete catalog online and order directly with a credit card (**www.keats.com**) or request a sample catalog by email (**order@keats.com**)

☞ Fax your request to **(203) 972-3991**

Keats Publishing, Inc.,Customer Service, Department 1
27 Pine Street, Box 876, New Canaan, CT 06840

Yes, *please send me a free Keats Publishing catalog.*

Name_____

Address _____

_____

City _____ State _____ ZIP Code _____

Do you know someone else who may be interested?

Name_____

Address _____

_____

City _____ State _____ ZIP Code _____

Optimum Wellness
The Information You Need
For Responsible Self-Care

Each issue of *Optimum Wellness* contains an unbeatable combination of the latest health issues written by some of the leading names in the alternative and complementary medicine fields. Four times a year, it brings you six informative pages on the most exciting and health-saving breakthroughs and products needed for maintaining, protecting and enhancing your health. Health professionals such as Kilmer S. McCully, M.D., Jeffrey S. Bland, Ph.D. and Susan M. Lark, M.D. are just a few of the authors whose contributions have made this newsletter a fantastic tool. We think you will agree this newsletter is the beginning of the path to optimum wellness.

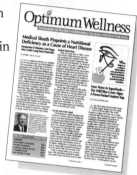

Just complete and mail us the coupon below, and we will send you a sample copy of *Optimum Wellness* free of charge!

Keats Publishing, Inc., Customer Service Department 2,
27 Pine Street, Box 876, New Canaan, CT 06840

Yes, *I would like a complimentary copy of* Optimum Wellness
Please mail my free sample copy to:

Name _____

Address _____

_____

City _____ State ____ ZIP Code _____

Do you know someone who might enjoy *Optimum Wellness*? Give us their name and address and we will send a sample copy free!

Name _____

Address _____

_____

City _____ State ____ ZIP Code _____

* Request *Optimum Wellness* or a catalog or place an order for any Keats title on the Internet! **www.keats.com**